About my writing

I0423628

Health
Health from Life
Healing
Back to Health
Hands On Healing...
Meridians
Organs, Muscles, Articulations, and all those Places...
Distance Healing
Lovergy
Bifocal
Maintenance
Chakras
Treating A Patient
Recommended Tools

Workshops
Words
I write
Audio books
Training & Coaching

#alternative #condition #disease #energy #healing #health #ill #illness #medicine #natural #organic #skill

Health

#alternative #condition #disease #energy #healing #health #ill #illness #medicine #natural #organic #skill

Coming from a multinational multicultural family I learnt many languages and to deal with many cultures... I have also lived in a few countries...
This has shown me the importance of words and communication.

Words are sweet water to my lips...
For lack of a better word I'll make up my own if I have to... if it serves the purpose of my writing... words are all yet sometimes words are not enough...

From the minute I could write I wrote... on everything and anything I could find to write on... I wrote I wrote I wrote... and I haven't stopped writing yet...
My first memory of writing was at home writing my name on my little blackboard... My father came to correct it... and writing was on for me from that moment on...

There was a time poetry belonged in popular culture before it was held hostage by the elite...
In many respects and ways I have long felt I belong in those days...
People quoted and cited lines from poems as people today sing along the streets...
And words were their music...

A couple of years ago one of my students presented a piece of his work about Louise BENNETT -the first Jamaican woman poet- and he got me thinking on how I wish I could go back to the dawn of writing... to be the first person ever to write the first book in his language... the first fiction...
Or even... Bulgarian born Elias CANETTI who, from wanting so much to understand the private thoughts his parents shared in German, went on to become one of the greatest German writers of his time and beyond... because with writing comes history... and stories...

My main interests belong in life, people, communication and nature.
People usually don't see the surrealistic aspects of their life... when I do...

Most of my endeavours are about communication and my writings are very oral in fact... they are meant to be heard and said more than read... even if one should indeed enjoy reading them... whether books, texts, poems or songs would easily find their way to the radio or stage... and I have recorded a few that I offer for sale now...

I also write for business and communication as well as for children... in a style that blends fact and fiction as well as poetry and prose...

Most of my books come in French, Italian and in English.

#alternative #condition #disease #energy #healing #health #ill #illness #medicine #natural #organic #skill

Our brain and mind host a whole wealth of unsuspected skills and faculties that lie dormant in the midst of whatever we may scrape up together and use through the meagre training and experiencemost of us painstakingly collect through life…
Sadly most of those skills will never see the light of day and both society and the industry make sure they remain well hidden in the dark corners of our soul…

Every so often one of us is hit by a rude awakening and ermerge to reach those depths and resurface all the better for it… enriched with a new knowledge and awareness that challenge the hardest facts of life… like the fact that life and health are not what they're cracked to be but but better and have so much more to offer us… natural health and well-being a the touch of our fingertips… and some of this is what I intend to share with you here… how to get better and enjoy a better health and life…

I was lucky enough to understand from a very young age that your life is what you make it… and that the destiny of man was evolution… and to the willing heart there was no limit…

Being human means being evolutionary… Man is not meant to stay in his primary condition but to evolve again and again… this is what places him above all the animals…

Healing is one of those skills that make the human what he is… too often a forgotten skill left to some 'freaks' as though life was freakish… and human talents designed to benefit a mere chosen few…

We all have it in us to evolve and we have those talents… talents that link us to the world around us and the whole universe and beyond… energy is everywhere to be found because there is life in one form or another everywhere…

Whatever its form life is in motion… and life is energy… energy willing –waiting- to be set in motion for the greater good… energy within the reach of anyone ready to make the most of it…

A whole wealth of energy we're bathing in is all around us… at the ready to come to our rescue… for us to tap into…

In this book I will give all the keys to exercise your own health… and work your way back to health… with simple exercises and practice…

Health from Life

Many people suffer everywhere without ever finding solace in their quest to regain their health... and sadly the medical field doesn't bring a conclusive definite answer to the pains and pangs...

Alternative medicine often offers a more natural solution... but then again often until a relapse into a sorry condition...

If our doctors are trained to treat us and sworn into medicine on Hippocrates's oath... which promotes the return to health with all and any treatment available... the fact remains that they load us with chemical stuff that come with a whole array of undesirable side effects... offer requiring then intake of ore medicine to ward off the side effects of the latter !

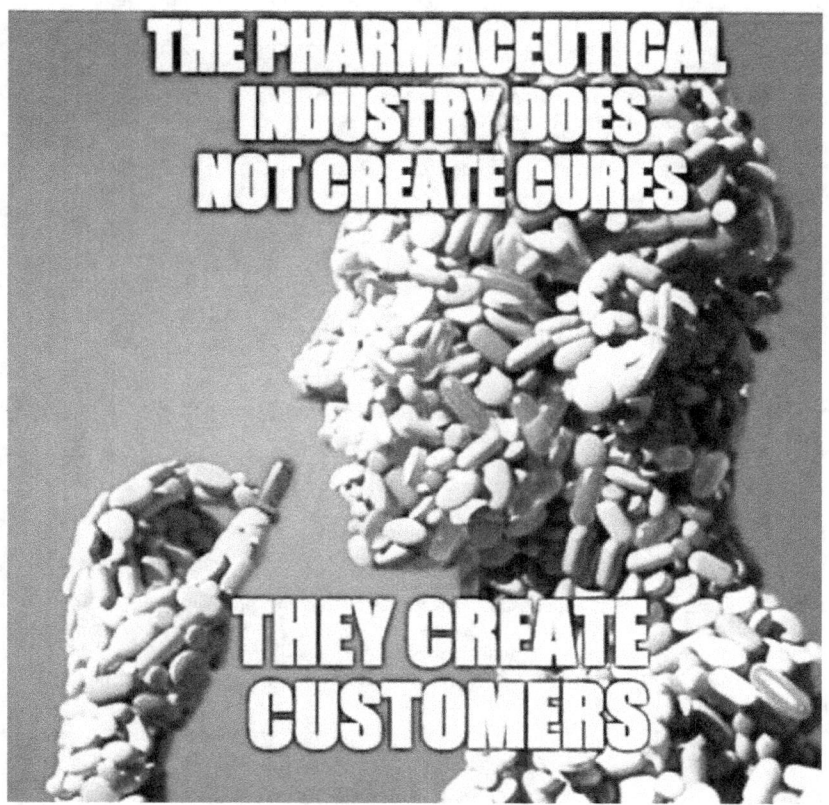

I mean by **healing** that the patient doesn't need to take any medication of any kind any linger... if not for life at the very least in the long run... the patient that has been cured does not take anymore treatment ever !

Ever since I have been cured I have not taken anything in the way of medication or treatment... not even for a headache !

Dietary supplements are only another form of addiction... if they might bring temporary relief... although most of them are a total waste of good time and money... they never cure anyone of anything... most of their customers end up forgetting about them sooner or later...
To bring any relief or cure, the patient would need to take tons of them... every day !
Chemical treatment bring massively powerful doses to bring a minimum result...

Sport doesn't mean shape... nor health come to that matter... quite the contrary !

If a little sport will take you along way on the path of shape and health, too much sport will kill you... suffice it to look at a regular sports person's X-Rays, Scanners and MRIs... and you will discover how broken they are all over ! Not to mention all the side effects and permanent damage caused to organs, muscles and tendons... beyond repair or therapy...
Bioenergy addresses those issues and bring relief and cure in a fast and efficient way... while effortless and painless... no pain yet all gain...

Believe it or not... but the hardest job you have probably ever done was your own **birth**... and probably the longest...
But birth is not without consequences neither for the mother nor for the child...

For the mother first who has born the baby all along with all the tremendous changes her body and metabolism have gone through...
And then the child... if everything revolves around him and adjusts to him inside... the child also suffers from movements and pressures...

Still... nothing to worry about... as bioenergy brings a soft and durable relief... affordable to anyone...

Bioenergy gathers all practices that use and promote the ambient energy available in the universe and beyond... towards the healing and improving of the health of all living beings... whether person, animal or plant...
Several arts are at the patient's and the practitioner's disposal such as Reiki, Chi Kong, Tai Chi and Prana Yoga to name but a few...
Just make sure you put yourself in the hands of a good practitioner...

Other **solutions** exist... other treatments are available in mother nature itself... and are both easy and within anyone's reach provided they learn a few facts and practise a few easy exercises...
Besides all this, dietary supplement remain expensive...

#alternative #condition #disease #energy #healing #health #ill #illness #medicine #natural #organic #skill

Most people still believe we live in 3 dimensions but truth of the matter is there are other dimensions most of them are not aware of... and energy is certainly one of them...

I have seen how a body can change many times... in hours... sometimes in minutes... from good to bad... and back from bad to good... many things can make our body change... whether weather conditions, genetics, age, activity, nutrition, or simply nothing... or nothing clear...
And we can help and make that body change in record time for the better...

This has shown me how our body not only is born and grows on to decay and die... it may also be moulded and shaped and be made to obey our will...

Many tools offer better health or promote a better lifestyle leading to better health... the sad thing is most of them offer no tangible results... or so little... and that at the expenses of drinking or eating tons of stuff we don't like and don't enjoy... or doing taxing unpleasant exercise for lack of which we might as well lie down and die... while other people are blessed with a life-long –and long life- of health free from pain and ailments... nature's way to remind us how different we can be...
Other people choose faith and go for faith healing... but, then again, not everyone seem to find a cure there...
I have tried many of them... all to no avail...

I come from a long line of severe physical conditions and ailments... my father often joked saying that he should have married a chemist... although he too took medicine all his too short life... and more than my mother at that ! And despite a life-long record of prescriptions his condition only worsened with time... he ended up dying at only 55... and after 2 strokes and many heart attacks...
While my brother has severe heart problems... my sisters seem to have been spared a life of toing and froing back and forth to surgeries and chemists... so far... and good luck to them...

I have long lost count of all the ailments that plagued me... one on top of the other... and next to the others... I have lost count of all the doctors I have seen... in a number of fields... all to no avail... I have lost count of all the alternative medicine practitioners I have been to in the hope of finding the solution... I have lost count of all the medicine and treatments I have taken... I have lost count of all the money I have paid and wasted... until I found my own answer... with energy healing I have worked my way back to health at last... and invite you to join me...

One thing is sure... we are not born equal when it comes to health...

I have had to watch my health all my life...
I am not a hypochondriac... I actually hate being sick and taking drugs... but I was always bothered by one thing or the other... as much as I hated it... desiring nothing more than a peaceful life... free from trouble... yet my expectations were to be met

#alternative #condition #disease #energy #healing #health #ill #illness #medicine #natural #organic #skill

by sorrow and pain... and an early declining condition... often calling death to my rescue... as all I ever wanted was my peaceful and quiet life...

In the summer of 2007 I woke up one day not able to move... or barely... I couldn't even turn in bed... I had to stay in bed all day... and the following weeks...

I went to see my GP after 2 weeks of unpaid sickness leave and hardly able to move... doing nothing but sleeping... and waking up only to fall asleep again... and told him I had been like this for a fortnight... and was sleeping day and night so tired I was...

That didn't worry him in the least and he told me he could be stress... stress ? In one fell swoop ? He gave me another 2 weeks' sickness leave... 4 months later things were almost as bad... he continued telling me it was stress... and did nothing more than give fortnight after fortnight of sickness leaves...

He did not recommend any test nor seeing a specialist...

Things remained the same until I talked to a colleague who is a shiatsu practitioner... and offered me a session that put me back on my feet in 20 minutes !

That's what traditional medicine is today... a waste of time and good money...

I eventually understood that I would get nowhere if I didn't ask for anything and insisted on seeing a number of various specialists and testing various things and functions... all to no avail...

Modern life has brought more trouble than solutions to our health... as if on one hand the medical field has made tremendous progress so have pollution and stress... to name but two... and if some of us take living to be older for granted today... a lot of our old folk now experience the problems of aging... decline and decay...

All that time I had been looking for relief that would free me from life-long chemical addiction and all its more than undesirable side effects...

Healing

Healing is the process by which the sick are permanently cured when their health is restored... until complete recovery... by one way or the other...
Doctors too often given us drugs that will have us addicted for the remainder of our days... too often benefitting drugs moguls more than suffering... while some low profile healers will work you back to health and regular life...

My whole life has been devoted to finding solutions to my problems and others' problems... and I long thought I would die trying...
I strove... asked and listened... tested and tried... hunted high and low... to no avail... for a long time... only left to strive on...
Some solutions brought me relief... for a while... and seemed to wear off... as time wore on... I seemed to be retracing my steps... backtracking to illness...

I studied relaxation, suggestopedia, hypnotherapy, music therapy... even saw a shrink for a while... every time one step closer... but never there yet...

From relaxation and yoga I went into sophrology... suggesting myself back to good health led me to a shrink... and for a wile I must confess I felt half way to paradise... hypnotherapy and music therapy came my way to complete the picture of better health... and took me to Reiki... Quantum Touch, Tai Chi, and eventually Chi Kong... And all the while people told me every time I touched them they felt instantly better... and maybe that helped my romantic life too... yet I was still intent on my *No Pain No Gain* education...

Until I fell into another dimension... until I found myself faced with another reality... reality comes in a whole array of shapes and ways... and there is much more than meets the eye to reality... or realities as it should be more appropriately coined...

#alternative #condition #disease #energy #healing #health #ill #illness #medicine #natural #organic #skill

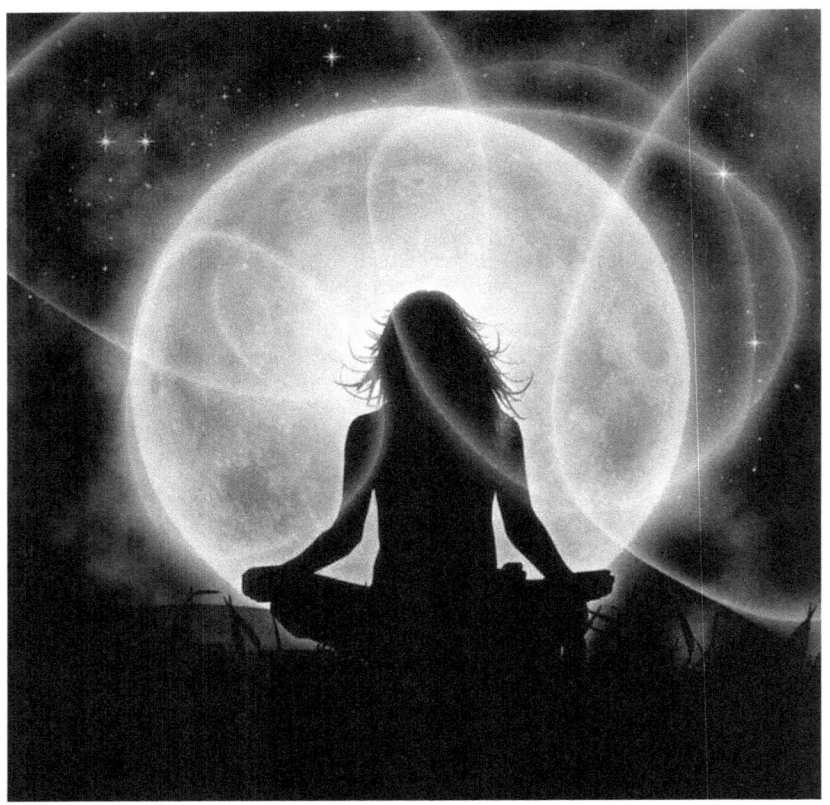

Energy Going... Going Energy...

One of my exes kept telling me how good she suddenly felt the minute I put my arms round her shoulders... and a colleague in excruciating pain told me how good my hand felt on her painful arms...

I did some energy healing on a colleague... I was working on her head... not touching her... and she said she could feel things moving inside her head...

Until I finally realised that when I rested my hand on an aching part of my body... I too felt much better !

It all started one day while riding on a suburban train with a splitting headache... I relaxed and closed my eyes and began to see colour patches waltzing behind my eyes and relaxing me... while I could feel the pain wane... and eventually go away... back home I enjoyed a good and healthy evening...

#alternative #condition #disease #energy #healing #health #ill #illness #medicine #natural #organic #skill

Later I realised I was systematically put my hand to cover a part of my body that was painful then... and in a jiffy the pain had gone... but gone where ?

Energy is the spice of life... and is found everywhere and anywhere... all we really need to do is to learn to welcome it and steer it... healing with energy works like magic... we just find the energy we need on the premises... and it is begging for action !

A pain or an ailment is usually no more than a lack of energy in our metabolism and surrounding... once it's found and put in the right place it begins its restoring work... put energy around you to good use... energy is always on the go and will getting you going... or going again... get your energy going for you !

What's more positive energy attracts positive energy...

Believe it or not our body is ready and willing to change for the better... and all it takes is a little effort on our behalf...

#alternative #condition #disease #energy #healing #health #ill #illness #medicine #natural #organic #skill

I eventually found a way that could be used anywhere... was non invasive... worked on the body and soul... whether the patient believed it or not... I never leave home without it !

What's more... energy healing is non invasive...the patient doesn't need to believe in any special creed... doing anything other than live in particular... the patient doesn't need to eat or drink anything special... the patient doesn't need to under for treatment... and you will only lay your hands for a short time on a specific part of your patient's body...

Energy healing appeals to the body as much as the soul... and psychological aspects of our persona... all benefitting of the treatment...

And with energy healing... the giver benefits of the energy just like the receiver...

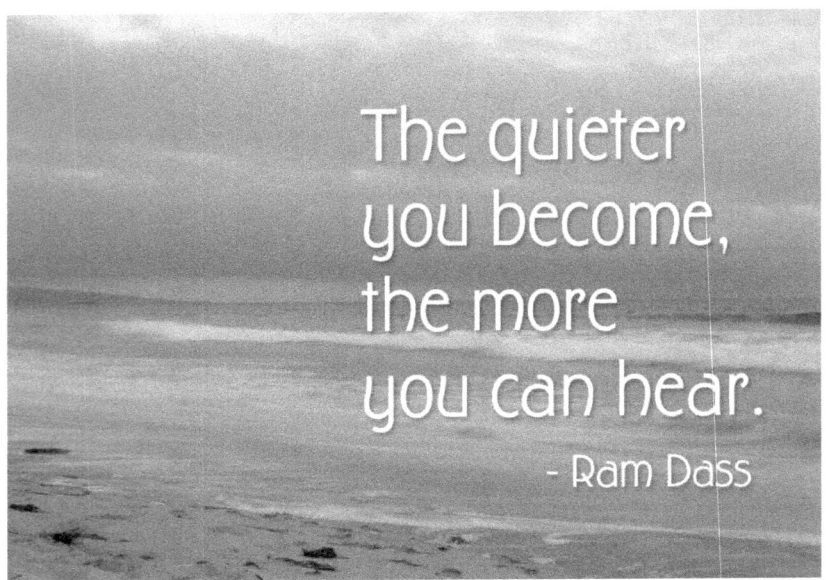

The quieter
you become,
the more
you can hear.
- Ram Dass

You will hear —and have probably already heard- from anything to everything about energy... often except the truth... while in actual fact you don't need to be an energy expert nor an energy engineer... all you need is to feel it and steer it... feel where and when it's needed and drive it back home... and you may do so in so many ways... few and far between...

Once you have mastered this skill, you're free to use it at will and wherever needed...

Andra's story

Andra was not happy... her busy hectic professional and personal life left too much to be desired... and only left her with a craving for a better life...

When she confided in me I told her about bioenergy and benefits it brings in many respects... and she agreed to try a session...

I proceeded to work around her head... as most of her stress came from managing her emotions... and then we would work on her heart...
I didn't touch her at all... no physical contact was involved... but she told me she could feel things moving in her head... and how she was becoming more and more relaxed... working her way back to complete relaxation and peace of mind...

Xavier's story

Xavier was very stressed... his life was shambles and falling to pieces at thirty-six... he could see no positive future for himself...

I asked him to lie on his sofa and check what was wrong to see how I could help...
With his eyes closed, my hand was scanning his body and the moment I hovered over his stomach he told me he could feel my hand... while I could feel his stomach begging for energy...
I then proceeded to give him a full energy refill in all that area and he was almost instantly relieved...

Nathalie's story

Nathalie would not come out of the dark... and remained with most of the lights turned off... all the time...
I asked her why and she answered she felt more comfortable that way as she had a splitting headache...
I looked at her and saw her face was that of a very old woman wrinkled with very big black rings and bags around and under her eyes... not the best description of the forty-five-year-old professional woman I knew...
I told her about bioenergy and Reiki... and how I could help her get rid of her migraine and relieve her in a few minutes... and she agreed...
Five minutes later she was a totally different woman... looking young and healthy again and her migraine had almost disappeared...

Nelly's story

Nelly, now forty-six, had had an operation on her forearm as a kid with a skin graft that had never left her alone... and the remaining cars did nothing to help her feel better... she told me she never wore short sleeves and cover her arm at the beach...
I came in to her office one snowy winter day and proceeded to give her energy... twenty centimetres away from her arm she told me she could feel the warmth from

#alternative #condition #disease #energy #healing #health #ill #illness #medicine #natural #organic #skill

my hand... to which I answered my hand was literally frozen from the cold still... and what she felt was my energy...

Nelly confessed she had never believed in energy treatment but within a few days I realised what progressed she'd made...

Alice's story

Alice doesn't know why for weeks he hasn't been able to breathe properly... and constantly snorts... round the clock... no treatment has helped so far... I only meet her every week at the office where she works...

When asked about bioenergy and reiki she admits to not knowing about them... and will try anything...

I offer to help with a few minutes reiki... and she gets ready for a three-minute treatment in between taking calls... every week her health gets better... until her condition is restored...

Farah's period pains

Farah is proud and happy to be a woman... if only it wasn't for those terrible period pains... she almost cries on the phone when I call her from Paris to Tehran...

We agree on a distance energy healing to take place on the spot...

She needs to leave her phone by her side on the loudspeaker... and follow my instructions...

She gets up again fifteen minutes later feeling relieved and pain free... better still her pains lessened in frequency and intensity... to eventually disappear after a few sessions...

Alannah's story

Otitis is murder when you feel your health is literally ready to explode from the splitting ear pain... especially when it starts at night when all doctors' surgeries are closed... and you live miles from the near hospital...

Alannah is on the phone barely making sense from the shooting pain's assault and any minute she'll shout down the line...

I tell her to lie on her bed and put the phone on loudspeaker...

She eventually relapses into deep sleep... and wakes up feeling fine the next day... still she couldn't believe energy could do this to her... and heal her !

Fakri's story

Fakri is one of my happy-go-lucky friend who seems to succeed in everything he undertakes...

He bought his first restaurant 25 years ago which still keeps being more and more popular and the same goes for the second one he opened over twelve years ago... and sitting at one of his tables he tells me he's opening a third one in a couple of weeks...

#alternative #condition #disease #energy #healing #health #ill #illness #medicine #natural #organic #skill

Fakri is the type of person who is always in a good mood whatever hits him... and life hasn't spared him either... he welcomes wall his clients with a heart-warming smile and hugs all his regular clients... the new ones soon come back too...

In the world of catering where staff comes and goes, most of Fakri staff have been loyal to him all along... and students who come to him for the summer holiday come back and sometimes even stay...

I am one to believe the biggest part of his success -besides the good food and service he provides- rests in the fact that people feel good in his company and the positive energy he radiates...

The best way to feel and get acquainted with energy is certainly to learn to relax... and lower your physical and intellectual activity to grinding to a halt... you may do this alone... or with music... Energy is very subtle... and you need to adjust to its level and tune in...

If you're one of those restless and fidgety people you may start by playing some music in the background as often and possible... and before long you will find a renewed inner peace... (check the music section further down)

Music is here to stay... and music therapy works wonders...

Jacob's story

Music will take you way beyond the furthest reaches of your imagination. I have a friend who has a young boy -Jacob- suffering Asperger's syndrome... he wouldn't go to school... was barely manageable... I worked with him prescribing certain music for two weeks... and we found him a different person much to his mother's surprise !
He became relaxed and manageable... more sociable... went back to school and wanted to study –even study music !- started making wonderful drawings for a kid his age and even grew in a matter of weeks !
I eventually rewarded him with an MP3 player for his newfound interest in music... which he has glued to his ears !

Katia's story

Katia confided in me one day that life at home was sheer hell... her two sons and her husband were nothing but bags of nerves and restless... all their negative energy bouncing back to her in full blow...

I told her about music therapy and asked her whether she would be ready to try... and she agreed... so I gave her my prescription... and let her go back home...
The following week Katia came back with a Cheshire cat grin right across her face... and told me how thankful she was... and how wonderful life was...
Life at home had become enjoyable again and the whole family was living in bliss... and her husband had even taken the music to his office...

Examples that go to show how much music can help you in your life and healing... for yourself... and for other people around you as well as your patients... just as much as energy... because music is energy too...
Use music during treatment and just sit back and watch the magic work...

Music will also enhance the efficiency of your work as a therapist and patient...

#alternative #condition #disease #energy #healing #health #ill #illness #medicine #natural #organic #skill

Hands On Healing...

Let us now look at the practical side of energy healing...

Let us go through the motion of energy... go with the flow... the universe is teeming with life and energy... you can't miss it...

To use energy healing, you will need to recognise energy around you, welcome that energy and apply it wherever and whenever needed...
This may not come naturally now to some people... but it is easy to pick up with a few simple exercises...
Anybody used to meditation and yoga may find this easier... but it is not necessary...

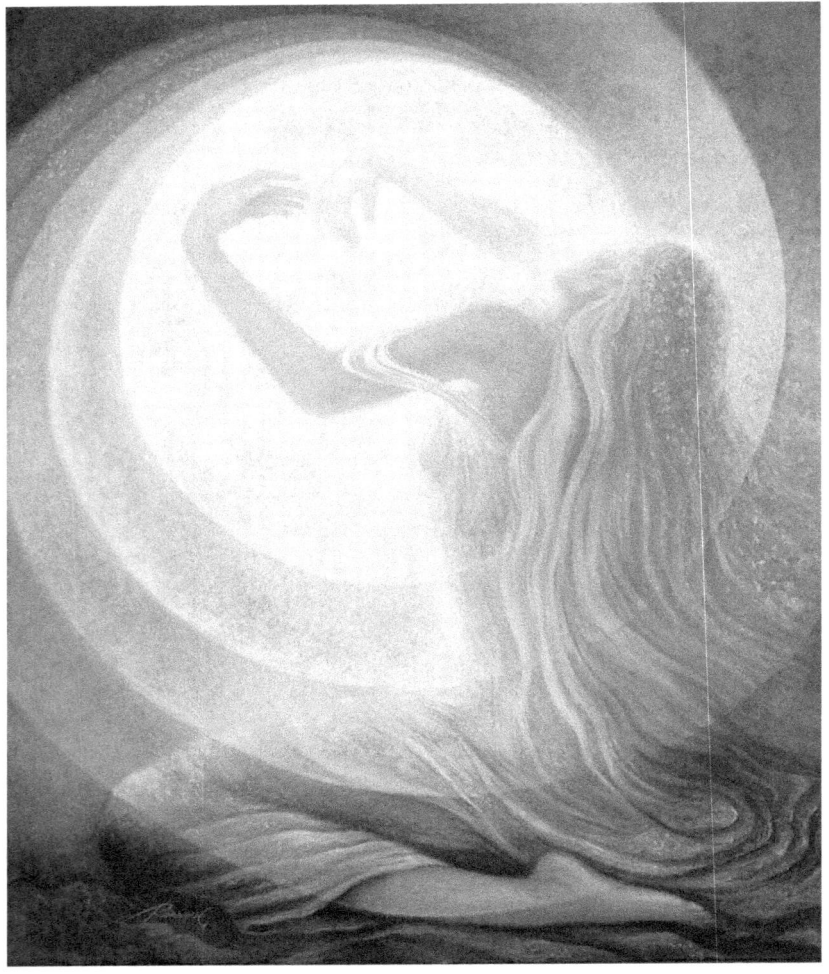

Welcome energy with life and love…

#alternative #condition #disease #energy #healing #health #ill #illness #medicine #natural #organic #skill

Cleansing

Before treating make sure you are cleansing the area to treat...

This is done by simply brushing over the pain with the hand or scooping bad or negative energy and sending it out to regenerate and return as positive energy...

This way a headache may be cured in seconds... just cleansing the head of the bad energy it has stored... often it's all that it takes !

Exercise One

This first exercise will enable to find your energy whenever you are whenever you need it…

Sit or lie in the dark… alone and undisturbed… and pay attention to the world and sounds around you… you may already feel some tingling or pressure points in your body already…
Try and hold the feeling for about 15 minutes…
And then let a light arise from under your feet and rise up to the top of your head very slowly… and let feelings and emotions come up with the light… making sure you are scanning you body bottom up and in a relaxed manner…

Do this for a week or more until the feelings become really clear… but don't expect too much at the beginning… you are not leading… you are letting go and welcoming without judging…

Exercise Two

This second exercise will enable to find or generate your energy whenever you are whenever you need it... which you may then use for energy treatment...

Once you sense energy you will need to welcome it and use it...

Sit comfortably and rub your hands together... when you feel your hands are getting warm... draw them apart very slowly until you can feel the energy pushing/pulling the hands to and from one another... the distance may be approximately 15 cm (5 inches)... but you will need to check your distance as it varies from person to person...

Practice this while continuing Exercise One for a week...

#alternative #condition #disease #energy #healing #health #ill #illness #medicine #natural #organic #skill

Exercise Three

This third exercise will teach you how to feel where the energy is missing and called for...

When you have completed and mastered Exercise Two... and your hands are full of energy... run one hand over the body of your patient at about 20 centimetres (approx. 7 inches)... very slowly... 'listening' to your hand... scanning the patient until you feel a tingling or being attracted to a particular part of the body... an energy vacuum begging to be filled...

Practice this while continuing Exercises One and Two for a week...

Exercise Four

This fourth exercise will enable you to begin the energy treatment of your patient...

When you have completed Exercises One to Three you can attract surrounding energy and manifest enough energy in your hands to start treating patients...

All the energy you will use is benevolent... so you have nothing to fear... all that energy will be good not only for your patients but for you... as the energy also runs through you and give you energy too...

You need to feel the energy around you... and collect it in your hands as seen above and start feeling the energy vacuum in your patient... and now leave your hands above the vacuum or directly on the part of the body calling for energy and let it flow in... to restore the natural operation of the metabolism...

And it doesn't stop there ! The energy you have place there for a reload... is only beginning to work and continue henceforth...

Furthermore, the excess energy –if any- will go treat the part of the body that needs it...

A good sign the energy is beginning to work is when you –and/or your patient- feel compelled to draw a deep breath... as though of relief... but this time of release...

Hold the position and feel the energy run for 10 to 15 minutes... the patient need not feel the energy although you most probably would feel it for it to work... it will work anyway...

Remember energy flows all the time in the universe without us being aware of its great work... and yet it works !

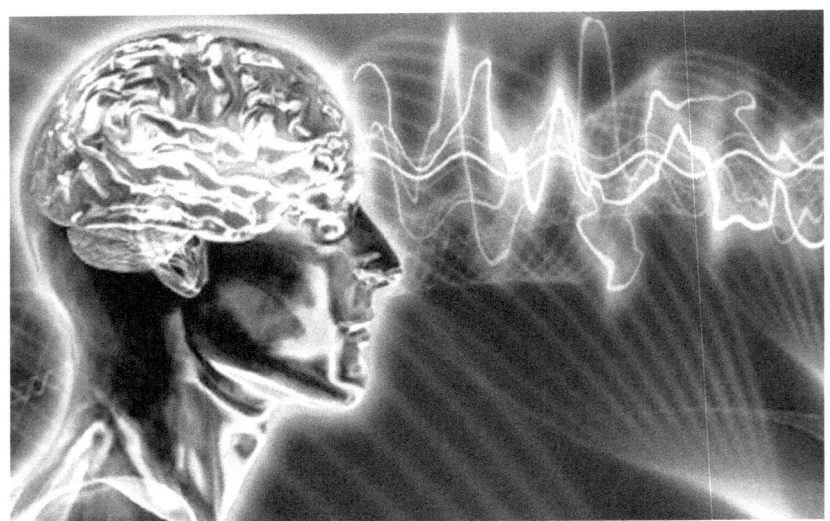

One or two hands ?

You may use one hand to heal with energy...
You may use both hands either side by side or in a sandwich position... or even on top of another... to treat an ailing area... often the energy intuition will guide you...
Treating with one hand on top of the other enhances energy in a particular area... it is also very good while treating small areas such as an eye for instance...

Practise as much as needed and as often as possible...
Energy healing works up a snowball effect... and the more you practise the better at it you get... and the better and quicker the results !

Meridians

Often while treating a part of the body you will feel and/or the patient will feel a tingling or pain in a totally different and distant part of your body the patient's body... that is because you have reached a meridian... as they are known in Chinese medicine... and the reaction is running all through the meridian to its end...

The meridian -or meridians- may also be put to good effect in an energy treatment... to supplement or substitute other approaches... all for the greater good and benefit of the patient...

Just place your hand(s) on the meridian and operate as per usual... and the energy will run along that meridian...

Organs, Muscles, Articulations, and all those Places...

You may be working on a particular area or part of your patient's body... or a particular organ, muscle, articulations or else...

In any case you will need to proceed all the same... in the same fashion... The stress and strain of the day may take your health away... but sometimes while looking for better health we overtax our body... and do more harm than good... and seriously damage parts of our body... tennis elbows are common in tennis players and athlete's feet are no only found in athletes...

I usually recommend maintenance to people who are prone to overdoing it with sports...

Distance Healing

You may need a phone call do this... and ask the patient to cooperate and relay your work... while you will operate as you would if your patient were next to you...

Make sure your patient is lying down and remains undisturbed during the treatment...

Lovergy

What better energy treatment can you give or receive but from a loved one ?

It is common in a family, especially with young children or toddlers to find one suddenly feels a pain, falls, or falls ill... or even maybe just feels tired or low down...

Giving and receiving energy can be a precious moment in a couple or a family's life... and one of the best...
What's more... treatment is always at hand...
Love flows naturally between people who love each other and kin... who often forget it and tend to be at the longest receiving end...

I strongly recommend regular massages and energy exchanges... particular in such trying moments as pregnancy, examinations, job hunt, ...

Bifocal

For the most experienced maybe... it is possible to treat two areas or pains or patients...

Life's energy is so abundant that it enables healers to do that !
Just apply treatment as learnt only focussing on the two parts or parties...

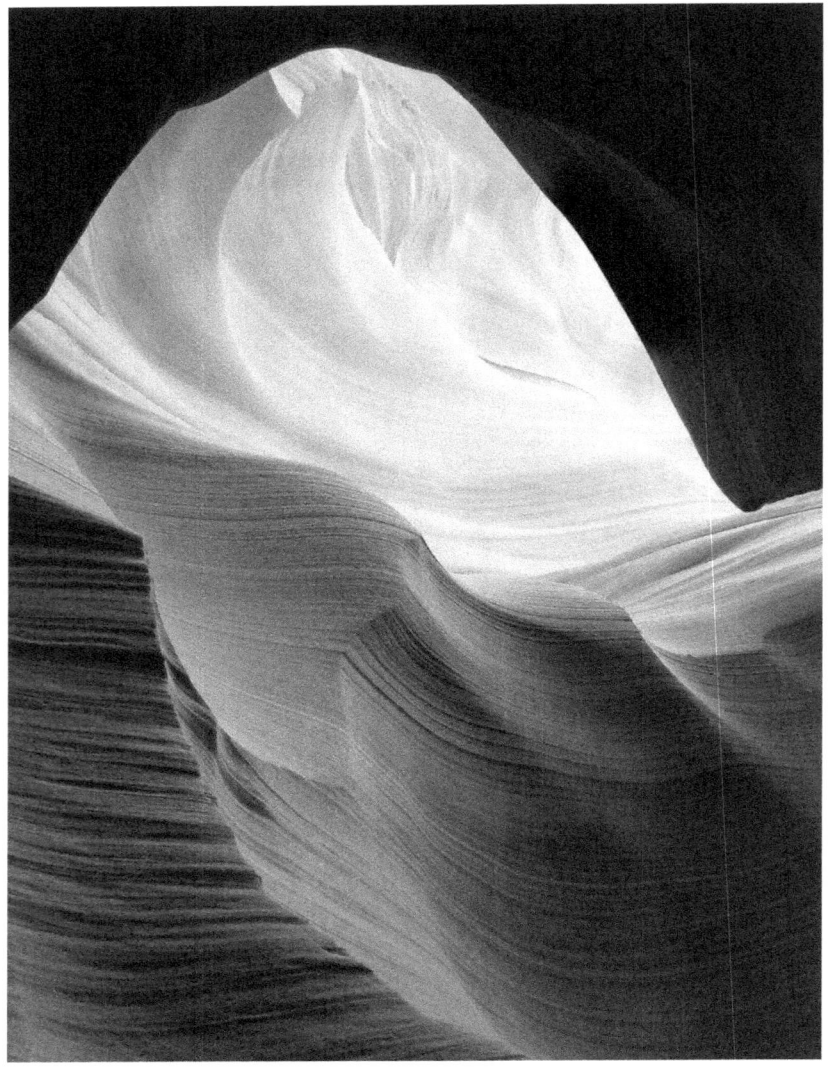

Maintenance

Like any machine, our body, our metabolism, needs to be maintained from time to time...

#alternative #condition #disease #energy #healing #health #ill #illness #medicine #natural #organic #skill

Maintenance because we wear and tear... and live all sorts of experiences and accident however minor and harmless they may seem... just like an automobile...

A good way to maintain health and energy is to give it a booster shot every now and then...

The best place to start is the chakras... as the chakras are literally the energy centres of the body...

Our bodies undergo wear and tear... and needs repairs... every now and then...

Chakras

The chakras are seven wheels of energy stretching along our spine... from the top of the head to the bottom of the spine... and each of them is dedicated to a specific area of our body...
The number of chakra will depend on the approach and healer... I remain loyal to our seven spine chakras... but feel free to work on the other chakras too...

When we give a chakra energy we boost all the parts to which that chakra is dedicated... promoting health alongside...

Energy treatment on chakras may supplement or even substitute an energy treatment session... and helps boosting lazy metabolism while ticking our whole body over...

Treating A Patient

Relax

To supply the best energy treatment and healing to your patient... have your patient relax...
Ask your patient to lie down... and relax him/her entirely...

Ask your patient to take 3 deep slow long breaths... and resume regular breathing...

After that ask your patients to relax their body progressively... and part after part... from the tips of their toes to the top of the head... telling the patient which part is relaxing and releasing tensions... relaxing... relaxing more and more... relaxing deeper and deeper every time you breathe out ... as you proceed with the relaxation until the whole body is fully relaxed...

Treat

Ask the patient what ailment or condition has brought him/her to you... and scan the part(s) with your hand at a distance from the body that may vary from 1 to 10 inches as it may be different depending on patient, healer or ailment... until you feel the area that is really pulling and begging for energy... cleanse the area to treat of its negative or worn energy and start treating that particular part or area... and start restore energy and health in the ailing zones, on the meridians and chakras... as seen in the exercises above...
You will treat with energy by restoring the part of the patient's body that is ailing... by channelling energy through you into the ailing part... and asking the energy to cleanse, restore and strengthen that part... as nature intended it originally...
Remember... **energy flows where attention goes**...

The patient may feel something or nothing during the treatment... that will not alter the effect... if your patients chose to talk and tell you what and how they feel welcome their feedback... but keep focussed... and apply until you don't feel the energy vacuum any longer...

One sure indicator that the energy is moving in is when you see the patient suddenly take a deep breath and relax deeper... the same happen to the healer most of the times...

Remember that to give energy treatment you need to enjoy and love what you do and feel positive... where attention goes energy flows...
Likewise your patient will need to trust your treatment... treatment requires two-way trust...

Time and experience have taught me never to treat who tell me '*I don't believe in it*'... those people will turn the energy you're giving them away... and prove you wrong... don't bother, you have nothing to prove to anyone...

#alternative #condition #disease #energy #healing #health #ill #illness #medicine #natural #organic #skill

Still you may send energy to people who are not aware of it... preferable at their bedtime...

Everybody and anybody may benefit from energy treatment... at any time... if they cooperate...

Musique Maestro, Please !

Music reaches the parts other treatment cannot reach... the vibrations in music move and shake the vibrations that reside in our make-up... and even rearrange them for the best effect on our body and soul...

Music therapy addresses and promotes better being and awakening... and yet most people –and even those who play and/or listen to a lot of music- ignore this and will only realise it through music therapy...

You may play some music during the treatment to relax both patient and healer... or for the soul pleasure of listening to music while you work...

You will find a list further down...

The number of sessions required will vary from patient to patient and ailment to ailment... but I have found that one session is usually enough... or treat in very short sessions which will raise the number of sessions...

If more sessions are required, then offer more... until healing is achieved...

Recommended Tools

Room

You'll need a room where you can accommodate your patients that will be quiet... and dimly lit...

Table

Obviously you will need a good table to treat your patients...

Cushion and blanket

A cushion may make your patient feel more comfortable in some positions... while a blanket may keep him/her warm during the treatment... as our bodies tend to lower their temperature when in relax mode...

Music

You may choose from a large span of music provided it is down-tempo...
My choice goes for such people as
- Sheila CHANDRA
- Frederic CHOPIN
- Dakota Suite
- Stephen HALPERN
- Eleni KARAINDROU (Ulysses' Gaze)
- Kitaro
- Robert MIRABAL
- R Carlos NAKKAI
- Arvo PÄRT
- Joanne SHENANDOAH
- Tanya TAGAQ
- Tangerine Dream
- Tata YAMASHITA
- Vangelis
- Antonio VIVALDI
- Mary YOUNGBLOOD

Native American Indian is always one of my first choices followed by synthesizer and classical music... make sure you find the music that literally resonates with you from deep within... although I regularly spend a day listening to Kattajait (Inuit throat singing)...
Explore music and experiment with your treatments... to find out which one works for you...

#alternative #condition #disease #energy #healing #health #ill #illness #medicine #natural #organic #skill

Workshops

I hold workshops in most places... to meet and further training with budding healers...

contact me :
jesse.craignou@yahoo.fr

Words

Words have always been -and will always be- a major part of my life…

The moment I could read I read… and the moment I could write I wrote…
Words have always exercised that magic on me... and words more than anything or anyone have opened doors for me… more than anything or anyone could have…

Words has a music of their own… Words will never let you down…

I write…
I write come what may…
I write whatever…
I write whenever…
I write wherever…
I write…

I wrote… before I could even write…

As soon as I put pen to paper, the first word is followed by another and another and another… and words tag on together… one after the other… and the words become my words for my greatest pleasure…
Words and I are words of a feather…

I look at my writing in more of an oral approach… spoken word's the written word here… our lips are not sealed… all in an introspective narrative spiralling style…

My writing evolves around not only words and ideas but also reason and rhymes… sounds like poetry… imagine you're listening… and let yourself be carried away…
My words depict the surreal side of everyday life… with all its eerie magic… riding the crest of the jagged edge between fact and fiction…

The music of my words is my melody…

Play on words play with words… play on sounds play with sounds…

Adaptations, articles, books, lyrics, musicals, poetry, reviews, scenarios, short stories, songs, texts, …

#alternative #condition #disease #energy #healing #health #ill #illness #medicine #natural #organic #skill

I write

Healing with Life's Energy is one of my books among which:

Pedagogical and business
Stories For English (also an audiobook read by Tory L. WILSON)
Stories For English (Student's Edition) (also an audiobook read by Dave WRIGHT)
Stories For English (Exercise And Practice)
More Stories For English (also an audiobook read by Kathy BRODERICK)
Stories For French
Singin' To English
The Comprehensive Teacher (Teacher's Edition) (also an audiobook read by Maxine LENNON)
Business English Test
English Tenses & Grammar (Teacher & Student's Edition)
Paris Passion
Finger Licking Good (also an audiobook read by Bobby BRILL)
Plain Sailing

Books and eBooks
Live To Tell
Righter (also an audiobook read by Maxine LENNON)
BioHazard (also an audio book read by David GEORGE)
A Woman's Day
Booster Shot (also an audio book read by David GEORGE)
Keeping Me Company (also an audiobook read by Helen LLOYD)
In Between Stations
Love Wars
Ten A Penny
Second Helpings
Visionary Mountains (also an audiobook read by Helen LLOYD)
Deflecting Patience
Umma Dawn – The Confidential Files
Redesigning Eden
At The Gaytes Of Heaven
Death Watch – A Matter Of Life
Love... And Stuff Like That !
To Think I Ran
My Greatest Hits
Poems & Songs
Quilled ! Words Of A Feather

Children stories (with Franklin ERDER)
The Alison Eating Monster
The Wolloes Have A Party
The Wolloes Go To Bed
The Little Stone Cutter

#alternative #condition #disease #energy #healing #health #ill #illness #medicine #natural #organic #skill

Audio books

Don't read much but ready to listen ?
Commuting ?

Try my audio books
Check Amazon, Audible & iTunes

Read by David GEORGE
BioHazard
Booster Shot

Read by Maxine LENNON
Righter
The Comprehensive Teacher

Read by Helen LLOYD
Keeping Me Company
Visionary Mountains

Read by Tory L. WILSON
Stories For English

Read by Dave WRIGHT
Stories For English (Student's Edition)

Read by Kathy BRODERICK
More Stories For English

Read by Bobby BRILL
Finger Licking Good

Read by Jesse CRAIGNOU
The Wolloes Have A Party
The Wolloes Go To Bed
To Think I Ran

Contact me: jesse.craignou@yahoo.fr

#alternative #condition #disease #energy #healing #health #ill #illness #medicine #natural #organic #skill